The DASH Diet:

A Quick Start Guide

by Dr. Terrell Clements

© 2013 by United Publishing House

Paperback Edition

ISBN 13: 9781499541366

The content of this book has been reviewed for accuracy. However, the author and publisher disclaim any liability for any damages, losses, or injuries that may result from the use or misuse of any product or information presented herein. It is the purchaser's responsibility to read and follow all instructions and warnings on all product labels.

For information, please contact the author by email at Authors@UnitedPublishingHouse.com.

Table of Contents

Introduction

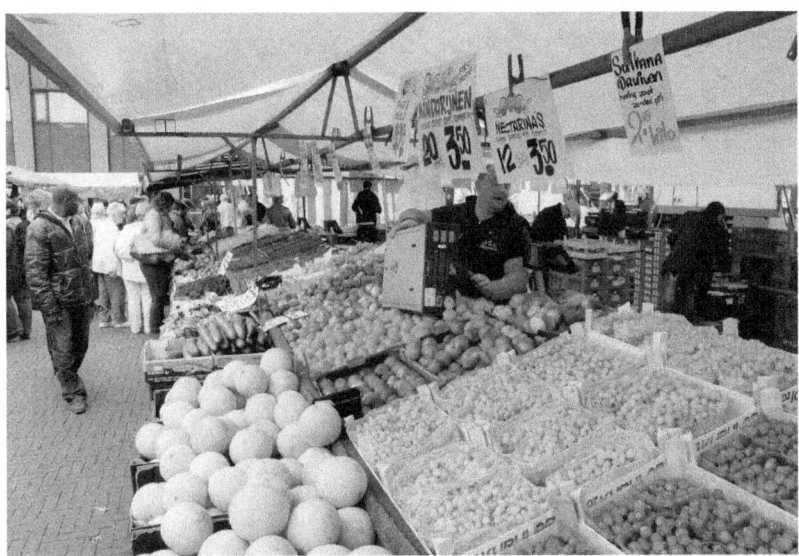

Hypertension and obesity are among the fatal conditions that affect many people around the globe. These conditions are typically prevalent among the adult population and are often caused by unhealthy eating habits. Individuals who suffer from these conditions are highly susceptible to fatal consequences such as heart attack. The mortality rate of these conditions is continually rising, alarming millions of adults and even teens. However, even if these conditions are extremely common and dangerous, they are also preventable.

Eating healthy foods is the best way to combat these conditions. When you eat healthy and avoid foods that are detrimental to your health, you will be less likely to suffer from a variety of medical conditions. In the end, it's more about knowing exactly what to and not to eat. Some people believe that taking medicines and pills is the best treatment for obesity, hypertension, diabetes, and other medical conditions. However, it is not at all true because as the old adage says, an ounce of prevention is always better than cure. The best medicine is actually following a healthy diet that can satisfy your body's needs.

The DASH diet is one of the most recognized and trusted solution to fight hypertension and weight gain. It is a healthy preventive measure against these conditions and is widely recognized as the best diet to resolve hypertension and obesity. There are several reasons why this heart-healthy diet is not just famous among dieters but also to nutrition experts. First, it is not unreasonably restrictive, and it provides the expected results just as long as the dieter consumes nutritious and low-sodium foods. It's also not costly since you are recommended to avoid processed foods, which are a bit expensive, and consume fruits and vegetables that are usually cheap.

This eBook will help you understand what the DASH diet is and how it can help you have a healthier body. You will learn how easy it is to prevent illness and to lose weight by just eating foods with the highest nutritional values.

What Is the DASH Diet?

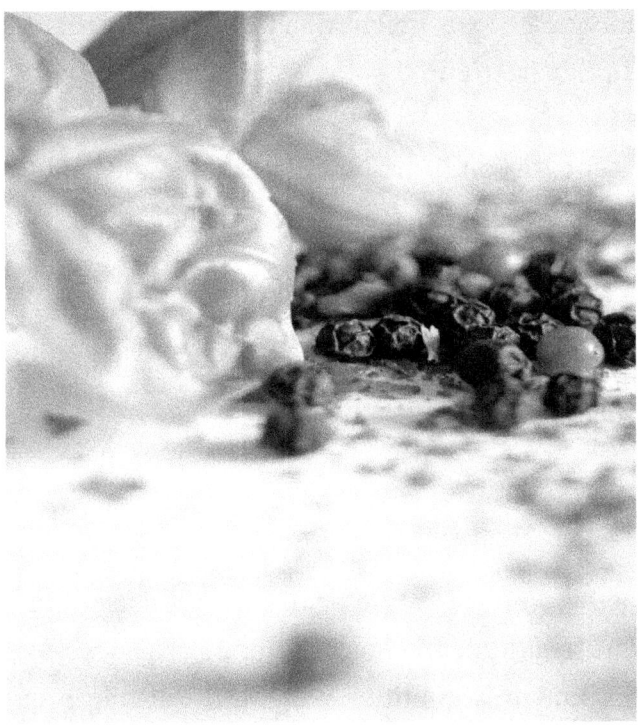

As the number of illnesses is continually rising due to the poor eating habits widely practiced by people, various types of dietary programs have also been developed. However, there is one exceptional dietary program that can truly help you become fit and healthier.

The DASH diet is a dietary program that is designed to prevent and control high blood pressure or hypertension. DASH stands for Dietary Approaches to Stop Hypertension, and it is composed of a balanced and flexible eating plan that is proven to reduce blood pressure. Individuals who are at risk of hypertension or those who already have it are highly advised to follow the DASH Diet. It is also known to help individuals lose weight due to the reduction of calorie intake in the program.

The diet focuses on heart-healthy eating plans and it highly recommends foods that are low in cholesterol, trans fat, and saturated fat. It also puts greater weight to the importance of eating foods that are rich in nutrients that can lower blood pressure. These nutrients include protein, fiber, calcium, potassium, and magnesium.

How It Works

It works by requiring a dieter to control his sodium intake and make healthy food choices. Dieters are urged to reduce their sodium consumption to below 2,300 mg a day. One needs to minimize intake of processed foods as they often contain sodium and other substances that can contribute to high blood pressure. The healthy foods recommended for this diet are vegetables, fruits, low-fat dairy foods, and whole grains. Hypertension is usually prevented or controlled by lowering sodium intake and increasing the consumption of healthier foods.

Why the Diet Emphasizes Reduction of Sodium Intake

The biggest risk factors of hypertension are a positive family history and weight and not sodium. However, sodium plays a major role in causing and aggravating the condition. If you are already suffering from hypertension, sodium will force your body to retain too much water in the blood vessels and make your heart work harder. When your heart's work load is excessive, the pressure in the artery walls will also increase, and this often results to high blood pressure. When you limit your sodium intake on a daily basis, it helps reduce your risk for hypertension.

Essential Nutrients Focused in the DASH Diet

Potassium

As mentioned above, sodium can cause and aggravate hypertension. However, you can fight the bad effects of sodium in your body through adequate potassium intake. Potassium works by stabilizing the negative effects of sodium. You need to take about 4,700 milligrams of potassium per day to lower blood pressure.

Magnesium

Magnesium can do many things to reduce blood pressure and prevent hypertension. It can help dilate blood vessels, keep your heart muscle and blood vessel walls safe from spasms, and dissolve blood clots.

Calcium

Calcium doesn't just take care of our bones and teeth but also our heart. It encourages normal vascular contraction and dilation that is essential to maintain healthy blood pressure levels. The heart is a muscle and it keeps beating normally because of calcium.

Folate

This B-complex vitamin can significantly help ease blood vessels, improve blood flow, and reduce the risk of hypertension. According to studies, people who follow a folate-rich diet are less likely to suffer from high blood pressure.

Fiber

According to researches, consumption of dietary fiber can also help reduce cholesterol levels and the risk of hypertension.

The fruits, vegetables, and other food items recommended by the diet contain plenty of nutrients. These nutrients can significantly help increase your immunity against illnesses aside from lowering your blood pressure.

The Science Behind the DASH Diet

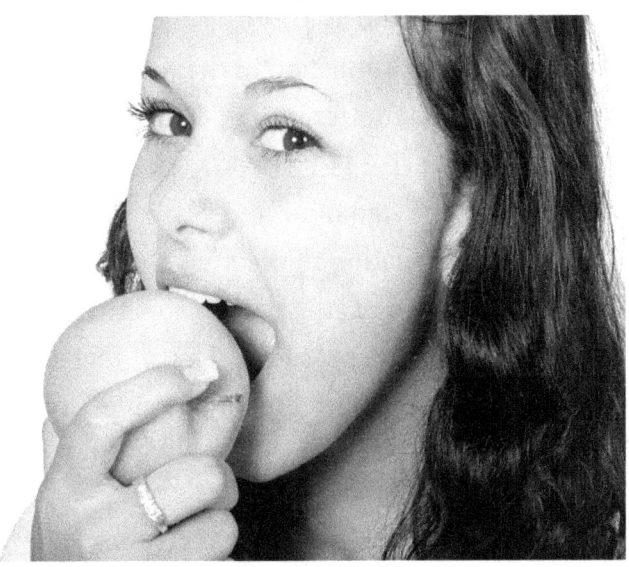

Dieters often need a proof in order to see how effective a dietary program is. If you are wondering whether the DASH diet is backed with studies to support its efficiency, take a look at these details to learn the science behind the diet.

The DASH diet has some strong science behind it especially if it's compared to many other heart-healthy dietary programs. According to researches and clinical studies, it has the capacity to reduce systolic blood pressure by 12 points and diastolic pressure for up to 6 points. Further studies claimed that the diet can also reduce cholesterol levels for up to 7%. It also lowers amino acid homocysteine and LDL cholesterol, which are known to increase the risk of heart disease.

Scientific Studies that Support the DASH Diet

Obesity in Men and Women

A study that was published in the Journal of the Academy of Nutrition and Dietetics showed the efficiency of the diet. The subjects were 144 sedentary obese or overweight men and women who had hypertension and were not taking any medication. According to the study, those who followed the DASH diet and did exercise were able to lose 19 pounds and reduce their blood pressure. The other subjects who did not practice the DASH diet maintained their weight and high blood pressure.

Weight Loss in Teens

Although it was not originally designed for teen girls or weight loss, it can significantly help reduce fat absorption or the accumulation thereof. According to USA Today, the DASH diet is also a weight loss solution for teen girls. Girls who practiced a diet that is similar to DASH experienced very small increase in body mass index within 10 years. A follow-up research even confirmed the results of the previous study.

What Makes the DASH Diet the Best?

The DASH diet was recognized in the 2012 Best Diet Rankings as the best overall diet by the U.S. News & World Report. It is considered as the best diet based on certain diet ranking categories. The DASH diet can provide long-term diet success, in addition to being heart-healthy and easy to follow. They also believe that, overall, the DASH diet is more nutritionally balanced compared to other programs.

Is It Safe?

Following the diet is generally safe as it's more about eating foods with the highest nutritional values and avoiding those that are harmful to the body. Unlike other diets, it is not associated with any nutritional deficiency because the food restrictions are directed towards the harmful food types. However, if you are suffering from any medical condition, you need to see your healthcare provider first before starting the diet on your own.

How Easy Is It to Follow?

One of the best things about the DASH diet is that you are only required to give up sugary, fatty, and salty foods and not an entire food group. This makes the diet extremely easy to follow for a longer period of time. The diet also aims at helping you feel full longer, so it's not going to be like you are depriving yourself. There are major restrictions, and there are also recommended food substitutions. Having a low-sodium diet doesn't mean that all the food you will take will taste awful. The diet suggests that you use herbs and spices to enhance the taste, and eventually your taste buds will adjust to it.

There are quite a number of studies and testimonies that support the efficiency of the diet. This is one of the major reasons why a growing number of people are also following the diet.

Can I Lose Weight on the DASH Diet?

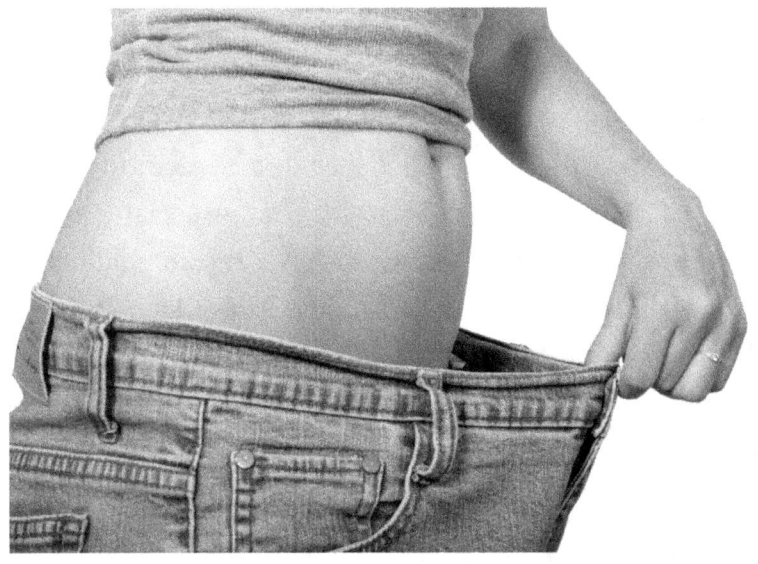

Losing weight is probably one of the most difficult things to do. There are different weight loss techniques that are already proven effective, and it includes the DASH diet.

As mentioned in the previous chapter, the DASH diet is designed to reduce blood pressure. However, you can also lose weight because the diet entails reducing your caloric intake. You can incorporate the diet with any weight loss program or strategy that you are using. The DASH diet recommends daily intake of health-promoting foods, but you should also ensure that you make low-calorie food choices. In addition to improving your eating habits, you also need to have an active and healthy lifestyle to lose weight.

How Does It Aid Weight Loss?

The DASH diet can help you lose weight by requiring you to have satisfying meals on a daily basis without overeating. It recommends nutritious foods such as calcium-rich dairy foods that are extremely beneficial for weight loss. According to researches, foods that are rich in dairy calcium can significantly reduce extra fat, especially in the waist areas of the body. You are also recommended to consume fruits and vegetables that are less in calorie as well as satiating protein-rich foods such as lean meat, fish, and poultry instead of meats high in fat. By avoiding unhealthy foods and consuming the ones with high nutritional value, you will be able to lose weight and have a healthier body.

Following the diet means that you need to reduce your sodium intake, or the amount of sodium levels in your body. You should also increase your intake of potassium, magnesium, fiber, calcium, and health-promoting nutrients. Doing this will not only lower your blood pressure, but will also help you lose weight.

How to Reduce Calorie Intake on a DASH Diet

You first need to determine the amount of calorie that you need to reduce. According to experts, if you reduce intake of 3,500 calories per week, you will lose 4 pounds after 1 month. You can gradually lose weight by simply taking fewer amounts of calories than the usual. You may list down all the best food choices that are low in calories and find out the amount of calories that each has. If you base your diet on the figure mentioned above, you may subtract the total amount with 500 to reduce your calorie intake to 3,500 per week.

There are different low-calorie DASH diet plans available, and they are the 1,200-, 1,600-, and 2,000-calorie per day diet. If you're having a hard time losing weight, you can choose the 1,200 calorie a day diet. If you just want to maintain your healthy weight, you can choose the 2,000-calorie plan. If you choose the 2,000-calorie diet, you are recommended to consume grains, preferably 6 to 8 servings every day. You should also eat 4 to 5 servings of fruits and vegetables on a daily basis. Choose low-fat or non-fat food and beverages to lower your calorie intake. You also need to reduce or eliminate consumption of high-fat foods such as fatty sweets, butter, cheese, and fried foods.

You will save 80 calories if you choose a medium-sized apple over four shortbread cookies. Instead of eating a hamburger with 6 ounces of meat, reduce it to 3 ounces and add a one-half cup of both carrots and spinach. This will allow you to save over 200 calories. If you are in the habit of consuming milk chocolate bars, eat a low-fat frozen yogurt instead to save 110 calories.

With the DASH diet, losing weight is not at all difficult mainly because it is not extremely restrictive. You just need to eat healthy foods with low calorie content and practice regular exercise.

Heart Health Benefits of the DASH Diet

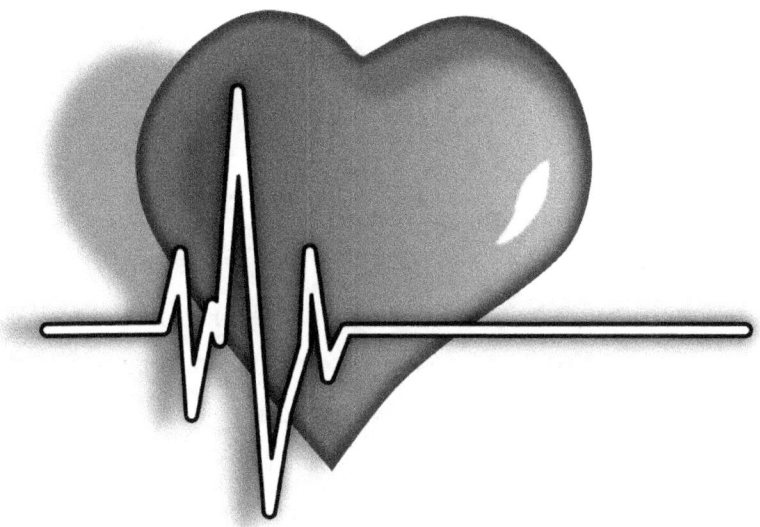

The heart health benefits offered by the DASH diet are one of the major reasons why it's extremely famous nowadays. Discover how the diet takes care of your heart more and protects it from fatal medical conditions.

Heart-Healthy Dieting Program

Almost all aspects of the DASH diet are heart healthy. Most people who are at risk or have cardiovascular problems are highly recommended to follow the diet. You may take a look at the reasons below and discover for yourself why the diet program is good for the heart.

It Recommends Fruits and Vegetables

These types of foods are loaded with vitamins and minerals that do not only make the heart healthier but also prevent it from having diseases. The foods recommended in this diet are rich in dietary fiber and low in calories and high-fat foods. Regular consumption of these foods can help you take care of your heart more.

Increased Intake of Whole Grains

The diet recommends intake of whole grains, and this can significantly reduce blood cholesterol levels and the risk of heart disease. Whole grains are excellent sources of heart-healthy nutrients. For instance, it recommends flaxseeds to be included in your meal plans. Ground flaxseeds are rich in omega-3 fatty acids and fiber and these can significantly lower your blood cholesterol levels.

Reduce or Limit Intake of Cholesterol and Unhealthy Fats

Following the diet also means limiting your intake of saturated and trans fats. These types of fat can dramatically increase plaque buildup in your arteries and this heightens your risk of cardiovascular problems and heart attack. When you follow the diet, you will be less likely to eat foods with trans fats and saturated fats; thus, you are less likely to suffer from heart-related problems.

Prevents Cardiovascular Diseases

There are certain cardiovascular problems that can be prevented and managed by simply following the diet. Take a look at the details below to see how the DASH diet can save you from these illnesses.

Coronary Heart Disease

It is common knowledge that high blood pressure can result to coronary heart disease. Hypertension forces the blood against the artery walls as the heart pumps blood, and if the blood pressure stays high over time, it can dramatically damage the heart and lead to cardiovascular illnesses. The DASH diet prevents this from happening by simply helping dieters to lower their blood pressure on a daily basis. It recommends foods that lower blood pressure, and thus, it reduces the risk of heart-related illnesses.

Chest Pain

Otherwise known as angina pectoris, chest pain takes place when the heart receives insufficient amounts of blood and oxygen. Plaque accumulates inside the coronary arteries due to high cholesterol levels, weight gain, and hypertension. The accumulation of plaque clogs the coronary arteries and deprives the heart muscle the amount of blood, nutrients, and oxygen it needs to function normally. The DASH diet reduces the risk of chest pain by recommending foods that lower cholesterol such as fruits with vitamin C. It also recommends consumption of garlic and onions that can also help reduce cholesterol levels.

Cardiomyopathy

Cardiomyopathy results from inadequate heart pumping. It takes place when the heart muscle weakens due to long-term high blood pressure and nutritional deficiencies, among others. The DASH diet can help prevent the development of the condition by recommending a reduction of salt intake that raises the blood pressure. It also recommends highly nutritious foods to combat nutritional deficiencies particularly of certain vitamins and minerals such as calcium and magnesium. Regular intake of these nutrients is highly recommended in the diet.

Individuals who are at risk or are already suffering from the condition can reap the best benefits by following the DASH diet. It satisfies the nutritional needs of your heart and body through the healthy foods that it recommends.

Additional Health Benefits of the DASH Diet

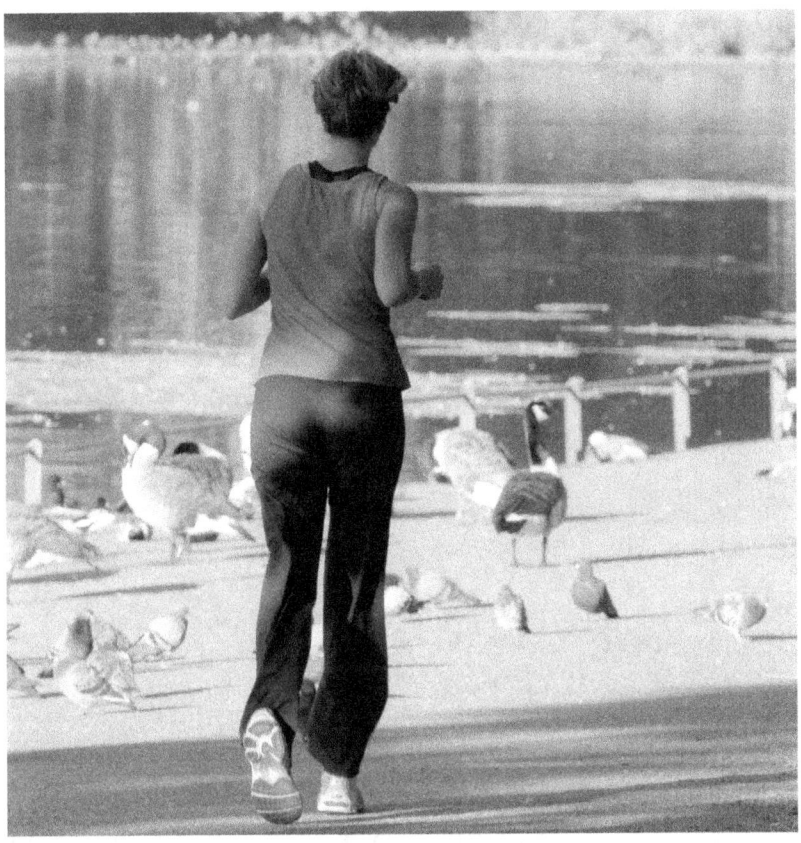

The DASH diet doesn't just help you take care of your heart but also of your other body parts. You may take a look at the details below to see how it can fight conditions such as obesity, osteoporosis, kidney stones, diabetes, and cancer.

Obesity

Being obese is extremely unhealthy and it makes you highly susceptible to a wide variety of medical conditions. When you follow the DASH diet, you can achieve the right weight and manage it to prevent yourself from gaining too much. It recommends consumption of foods that are low in calorie as well as limiting your sodium intake. Unhealthy food choices and eating habits are among the major causes of obesity. Excessive salt or sodium intake is also associated with dramatic weight gain. When you follow the DASH diet, you will be able to eliminate extra fat and manage your weight.

Osteoporosis

Studies show that excessive or unregulated salt intake can lead to osteoporosis. If you consume too much salt during adolescence, there is a great chance that you will suffer from osteoporosis later in life. These studies suggest that high salt diets increase urinary calcium secretion. If you consume salty foods, more calcium will be released in the urine. When you constantly consume foods with high salt content for extended periods, it would weaken your bones and result to osteoporosis. Since the DASH diet promotes reduction of salt intake and consumption of calcium-rich foods, it can reduce the risk of osteoporosis.

Kidney Stones

As mentioned in the above paragraph, excessive salt consumption can increase calcium excretion in the urine. When higher concentrations of calcium are combined with phosphorus and oxalate in the urine, it can result to the formation of kidney stones. Experts recommend the reduction of salt intake rather than your intake of calcium. The DASH diet prevents you from consuming foods high in salt on a daily basis but instead requires you to eat foods with fewer amounts of salt. By following the diet, you will be able to protect yourself from kidney stones without the need to lower your calcium intake.

Diabetes

Diabetes can develop from high blood pressure, high cholesterol levels, and obesity. The DASH diet works by preventing you from taking foods that can raise your cholesterol levels and blood pressure. It also helps you manage your weight and keeps you from becoming obese. The diet also ensures that you avoid too much intake of sugary foods. All these can significantly reduce the risk of diabetes. When you are on a DASH diet, you will be protected from the risk factors of diabetes and from developing the condition.

Cancer

Following the diet can help prevent the development of cancer. The diet promotes consumption of foods with the highest nutritional value such as fruits, vegetables, lean, meat, and whole grains. These foods are equipped with antioxidants, vitamins and minerals that can reduce the risk of cancer. For instance, nutrients such as magnesium and calcium can help reduce the risk of colon cancer. The diet also recommends the lower, if not zero, intake of processed foods, which are highly associated with the development of cancer.

You will not just avoid excessive weight gain and hypertension, but you will also be able to provide your body with long-term health benefits by following the DASH diet. You are allowed to eat quite a number of the healthiest foods available in the market. If you want to know what these foods are, check out the next chapter.

What Foods Are Included in the DASH Diet?

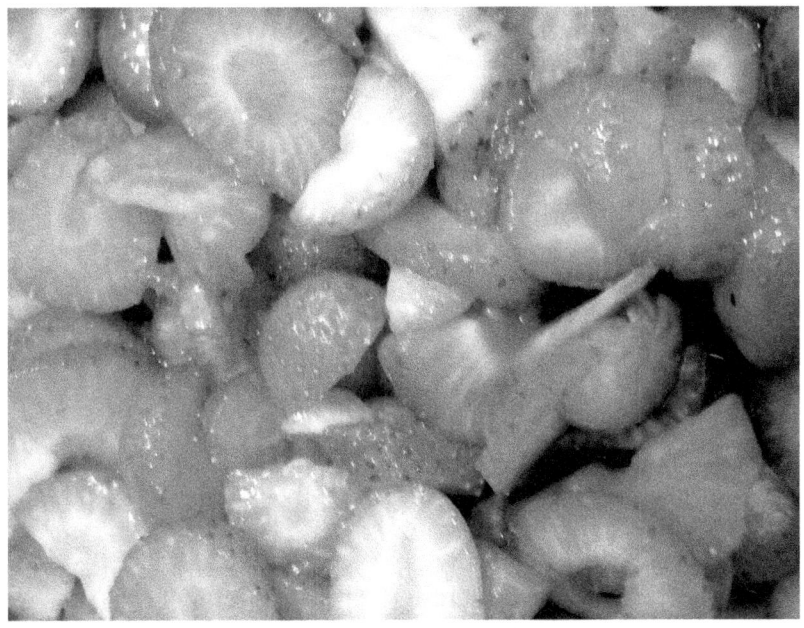

What you eat can have a dramatic impact on your overall health. In the DASH diet, you need to eat a wide variety of fruits, vegetables, and other nutritious food products. These foods typically contain potassium, magnesium, calcium, folate, and dietary fiber.

Fruits

Bananas, berries such as Hawthorne berries, watermelon, kiwis, apples, grapes, pears, pineapple, oranges, and avocado are among the best fruits recommended in the DASH diet. These fruits have powerful blood-pressure-lowering substances that can prevent and reverse hypertension. Bananas, for example, contain at least 450 milligrams of potassium. This amount can significantly offset the harmful effects of sodium. Avocado is another potassium powerhouse that also contains heart-healthy vitamins, phytonutrients, monounsaturated fat, and 975 milligrams of minerals.

Vegetables

Spinach is a fibrous green leafy delight that is low in calorie and rich in magnesium, folate, and potassium. These nutrients are extremely effective in lowering blood pressure. Kidney, Lima, navy, pinto, black and white beans as well as soybeans are rich in potassium, magnesium, and fiber. You can also include white, sweet, and purple potatoes in your list as they are also excellent sources of magnesium and potassium. Among the blood-pressure-lowering vegetables recommended in the diet includes artichokes, broccoli, cabbage, carrots, cauliflower, corn, mushrooms, lettuce, sprouts, squash, and mushrooms.

Meat & Seafood

Among the meat and seafood products included in the diet are beef, chicken, and turkey. According to studies, eating lean red meat can significantly help dilate the blood vessels and this results to low blood pressure. You should choose chicken or turkey breast and lean cuts of beef such as sirloin or tenderloin. Consumption of lean meat should be done in moderation. Salmon, herring, mackerel, shrimp, albacore tuna, and other seafoods that are rich in omega-3 fatty acids are also recommended because they can help reduce inflammation, cholesterol levels, and blood pressure.

Bread & Grains

Whole grains such as oatmeal, cereal, barley, brown rice, quinoa, whole rye, and buckwheat are also included in the diet. According to researches, whole grains have fiber, magnesium, folate, potassium, and nutrients that can help prevent hypertension. Whole wheat bread, tortillas, pasta, and wild rice are also recommended to people who follow this diet. Consumption of whole grains also aids weight control because they can make you feel full longer.

Nuts & Seeds

Certain nuts and seeds such as cashews, peanuts, pecans, pumpkin seeds, walnuts, almonds, hazelnuts, and unsalted sunflowers are also excellent sources of magnesium, potassium, and calcium. You may consume a handful of these edible items during snack time on a daily basis. Pistachios are also recommended because they are low in sodium and rich in heart-healthy monounsaturated fat.

Dairy Products

Low-fat dairy products are widely known to have nutrients such as potassium, magnesium, and calcium that can help produce and maintain a healthy blood pressure. Low-fat dairy products include reduced-fat cheeses, cottage cheese, margarine, sour cream, and fat-free yogurt. According to studies, people who consume 1,000 to 1,500 mg of calcium on a daily basis can reduce the risk of having hypertension. You can get calcium from food by simply consuming one or two cups of plain non-fat yogurt every day.

Herbs & Spices

Herbs and spices such as garlic, cayenne, onions, black haw, buckbean, hawthorn, Rauwolfia serpentina, and mistletoe are also included in the DASH diet. Garlic is an excellent source of medicinal properties that can significantly help reduce cholesterol levels, prevent blood clots, and relieve hypertension. Ginkgo biloba is also known for its capacity to dilate blood vessels and improve circulation.

Others

One of the recommended food items that you will surely love in this diet is dark chocolate. Just eat a small square of dark chocolate that contains 30 calories in a day. This will lower blood pressure in 18 weeks without weight gain. Raisins are also included in the diet because they contain more than 1,000 mg of potassium.

Beverages

Skim milk provides vitamin D and calcium that works together to lower blood pressure for up to 10 percent. Another recommended drink is red wine since it can prevent the onset of high blood pressure when taken in moderation. It can soothe the arteries and reduce your blood sugar level. For women, moderate consumption is one five-ounce glass per day and two glasses for men. Other beverages include hibiscus tea and grape juice.

There are many other food items that are also included in this diet. Most of them are also excellent sources of nutrients such as potassium and magnesium. In the next chapter, you will see the kinds of foods that you need to avoid and why you shouldn't consume them when following this diet program.

What Foods Should Be Avoided on the DASH Diet?

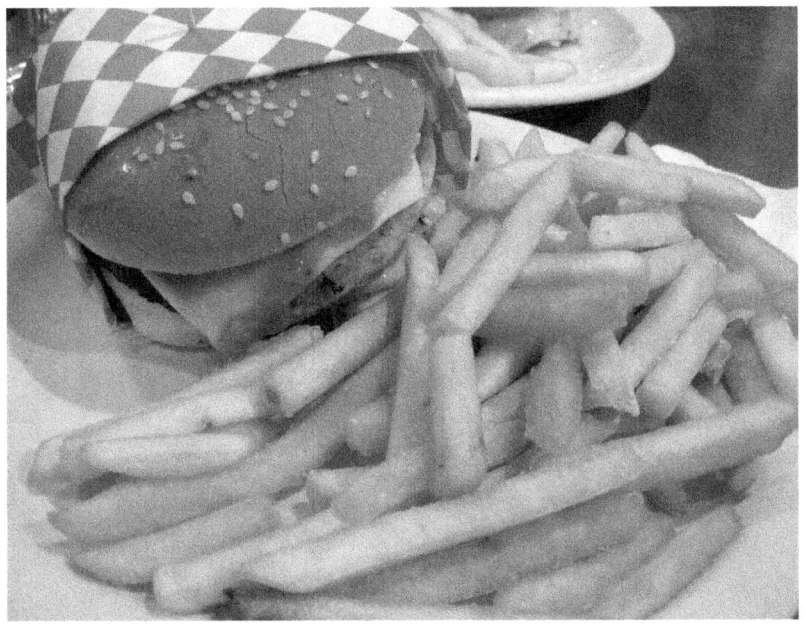

The DASH diet also discourages intake of various food items that are popular and available in the market today. Most of these items are considered by many people as an important part of their daily meals. However, these foods are extremely unhealthy, and they can cause irreversible damage to your body.

Salted Snack Foods

Salty snacks include pretzels, cheese puffs, tortilla chips, packaged nuts, and other junk foods. Although these snacks, especially pretzels, are often thought to be healthy because they are low in fat, you need to find other snack options because they're also rich in sodium.

Pizza

This is made from a variety of salty ingredients such as the cheese, dough, sauce, and processed meats. When you eat a slice of pizza, you may be taking an amount of sodium that's a lot more than the daily recommended dose. It also contains saturated fat that can contribute to weight gain.

Chinese Foods

Most Chinese dishes are extremely delicious, but they are also loaded with salt. For instance, one dish is prepared using a combination of Teriyaki sauce and soy sauce. A table spoon of these ingredients can actually contain about 1,000 mg of sodium.

Processed Meats

Luncheon meats, bacon, ham, sausage, salami, and hotdogs are not just loaded with chemical preservatives but also with sodium. According to studies, you are at lesser risk of having hypertension if you limit yourself from eating processed meats, just one serving per week or less will probably do.

Canned Goods

The DASH diet discourages consumption of any canned fruits and vegetables as they typically contain enormous amounts of sodium, sugar, or some other preservative. They also have sauces and seasonings that also contain great amounts of salt. Canned fruit juice should also be avoided since the process of canning raises its sodium level.

Fast Food Items

People who follow the DASH diet should also avoid French fries, sandwiches, burgers, and chicken tenders from fast food chains. A small piece of your favorite fries can contain up to 250 mg of sodium. This could be more if you consume frozen French fries. Most fast food chains offer sandwiches and burgers that contain over 1,500 mg of sodium. Chicken tenders, on the other hand, can contain 2,100 mg of sodium.

Instant Noodles and Soups

Instant noodles contain high amounts of food additives, flavor enhancers, preservatives, and sodium. Research shows that quite a number of instant noodles contain over 1,000 mg of sodium. You also need to reduce consumption of instant soups and stock cubes because they also have high sodium content.

Pickled Foods

Pickled foods and papads utilize high amounts of salt to increase their shelf lives. An average-sized pickle can contain 570 mg of sodium and this totally exceeds your daily sodium limit. When you consume 100 grams of pickled olives, you will get 1,556 mg of sodium.

Saltwater Crab

This seafood is a great source of omega-3 fatty acids and vitamin B12. However, you should consume it in moderation because it has high sodium content. If you consume 100 grams of saltwater crab, you will get 1,072 mg of sodium.

Sugar-Sweetened Beverages

Sugar can elevate blood pressure by making the blood viscous and the heart pump harder. You need to avoid sugar-sweetened beverages such as fruit punch, iced tea, and soft drinks. Fructose can also raise blood pressure and is normally used as an ingredient in sports drinks, pop, and flavored water. Sugar only acts as a sweetener, and it only has little nutritive value. When you are following this diet, you need to reduce or avoid consumption of these beverages.

If taking any of the foods above is part of your daily eating routine, then it is best that you start to gradually reduce your intake until you can handle completely removing them from your diet.

How Do I Get Started with the DASH Diet?

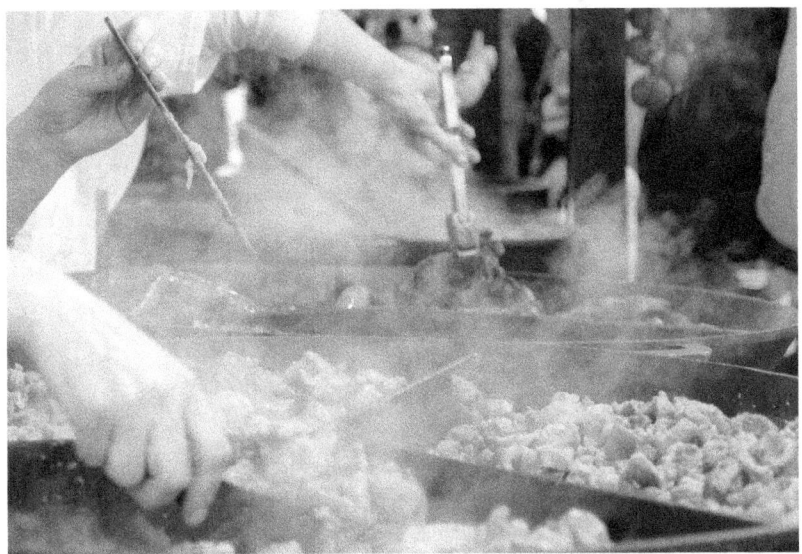

Starting the diet in the right manner is one of the most important steps that you need to take. There are several things that you should do to ensure that you are following the DASH diet in an appropriate way. Follow the essential steps below to properly start DASH dieting.

Read Food Nutrition Labels

This is one of the most important things that you need to do when starting the DASH diet. You need to know exactly what ingredients are contained in the product as well as the amount of nutrients that it has. You may take note of the serving size, the total calories per serving, the overall fat content, and the essential vitamins and minerals that the product is equipped with. When you do, you will be able to keep track of the nutritional values that you get every time you eat.

Choose the Low-Calorie DASH Diet Plan for You

As mentioned in the previous chapters, there are three different low-calorie DASH diet plans to choose from. You can choose 1,200-calorie diet if you are trying to fight weight gain and hypertension. There are also other options, such as the 1,600- and 2,000-calorie diet plans. Choosing the right diet plan for you may depend on your goals or the purpose of your diet, as well as your body's condition. If you are already suffering from obesity and hypertension and you don't have an idea about what plan to choose, then it's best that you consult your nutritionist.

Learn How You Can Effectively Reduce Salt and Sodium Intake

Aside from avoiding the foods that have high amounts of salt or sodium, you still need to learn how you can reduce your intake of these substances in your day-to-day life. For instance, you can use spices or salt-free seasoning blends to add flavor to your dishes instead of using salt. If you can't help but consume canned tuna, then you can just rinse the fish with water to wash off the sodium. When eating out, simply ask how the foods are prepared and make a request to have salt-free dishes. There are many other things that you can do to lessen your salt and sodium intake. You just need to remember that there should be less salt in whatever food that you eat.

Start Making the Changes Little by Little

Start making changes to your eating habits in a gradual fashion. You may begin by adding a serving of vegetables to your meal or use fat-free dressings instead of ones that are full of fat. You may start limiting your meat intake and eat only lean meats. There are many other small changes that you can do to make the dieting process easy. You can eat fruits instead of junk foods for snacks or drink fat-free milk instead of soda or other sugary drinks.

Properly Practice the DASH Diet

Once you have already started making the dietary changes, you then need to bring it to a higher level. For instance, if you have already included vegetables in your daily diet, add a few more servings during lunch and dinner time. You also need to focus on eating foods that are less in sodium and rich in potassium, magnesium, calcium, folate, and dietary fiber. Eat healthy and avoid foods that are harmful to your health.

Learn How to Deal With Challenges and Setbacks

There are challenges that can make your dieting process harder and stop you from achieving your goals. You need to prepare yourself for these challenges and get back on track. Determine what's making the diet difficult to follow, deal with the challenge, and allow yourself to go back to the dieting process. Bear in mind that making too much change in a very short period is often the cause of these challenges. Do things one at a time and try to introduce your new food choices to your body in a gradual manner. Write down your meal plans, track the minutes or hours that you engage in physical activities each day, and reward yourself for the achievements, even the small ones, that you attain.

Once you follow the steps stated above, you will be able to start the diet without encountering too many challenges. The next chapter will show you the common mistakes that you should avoid in order to make your dieting experience easy and enjoyable.

Mistakes to Avoid When Beginning the DASH Diet

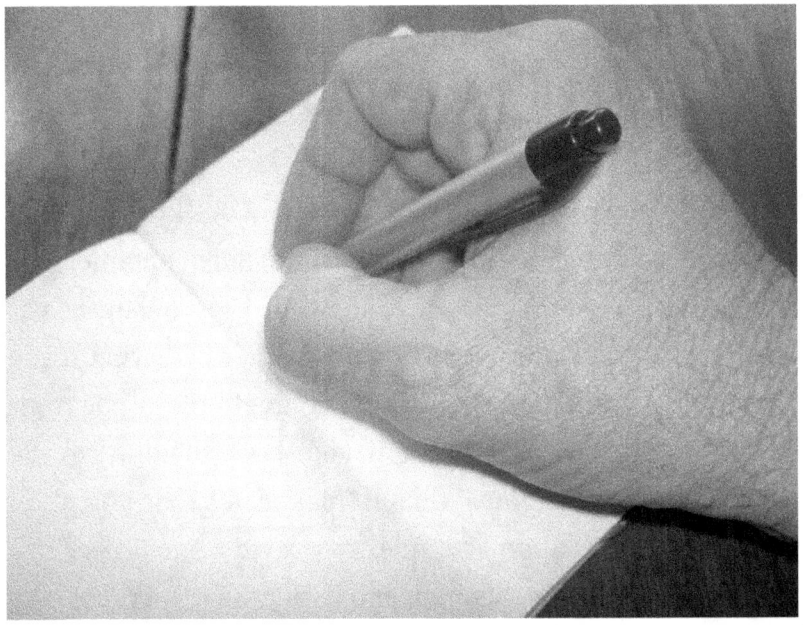

There are certain things that you need to avoid doing, especially when you are just starting the diet. Listed below are mistakes that most people often commit and that you need to avoid to reduce the challenges while dieting.

Shopping when Hungry

This is one of the common mistakes of dieters. They tend to shop while hungry and struggle about resisting high-sodium, high-fat foods mainly because everything looks appealing. Studies show that when a person skips lunch or breakfast before making grocery purchases, his brain easily reacts to fattening foods. Some people impulsively eat ice cream when they are starving while they shop. Make sure that you are not hungry while shopping to avoid the temptation of purchasing unhealthy foods.

Abruptly Making Big Dietary Changes

According to a clinical testing about the DASH diet, people who are not in the habit of eating fruits and vegetables can suffer from loose bowel movements if they abruptly eat these fresh food. You need to start the diet by eating these healthy foods in a gradual manner to avoid the unpleasant consequences. You need to allow your body to adjust to the changes until it becomes a habit. Make sure that you shop for enough fruits and vegetables to provide 2 to 3 servings for each person in the household per day. Increase the intake to 3 to 4 servings after a few days or weeks. If the dietary changes that you make are too much for you to handle, you will reduce your chance of achieving your goals.

Not Planning Your Weekly Meals

It is extremely important to focus on having the right food choices. However, you should not forget that planning your weekly meals is also essential. If you don't plan your meals, you will eventually find yourself not knowing what to eat when you're hungry. You might also not have the time to shop when this happens, so you will be tempted to consume fast food, which is the enemy of the DASH diet, because you're hungry. Bear in mind that one fast food meal can provide you with the amount of sodium that is more than what your body needs for two days. Plan your weekly meals to give you more time to shop for ingredients and prevent you from resorting to fast food chains.

Using Unhealthy Cooking Methods

Many dieters presume that all it takes to have healthy eating habits is to simply choose the right kind of foods. However, they fail to see that certain food preparation methods are extremely unhealthy over others. These cooking styles can significantly influence the nutritional values and calorie content of the meals. Lean meats, fruits, and vegetables can become unhealthy depending on how they are prepared. If you fry the food, it will be soaked in the oil and will obtain more calories. Boiling vegetables can also leach the nutrients into the water. Make sure that you use healthy cooking methods such as steaming and roasting. You can grill occasionally but just make sure you avoid carcinogens that can develop from charring the food.

Giving Up Easily

As mentioned in the previous chapter, you will be more likely to encounter certain challenges that will prevent you from reaching your goals. Some people easily give up when they encounter the challenges, and they often discontinue within days or weeks from starting the diet. You can stop dieting for a few days, and then try to get back on track.

Don't give up thinking that you can't do it as the trials that you are encountering are all part of your dieting progress. When you give up easily, you will end up jumping from one dietary program to another.

Many dieters discontinue what they have started mainly because they commit mistakes which they think can't be corrected. This negative mindset is yet another mistake that you need to avoid in order to start the dieting process smoothly.

Learning to Customize the DASH Diet for Your Needs

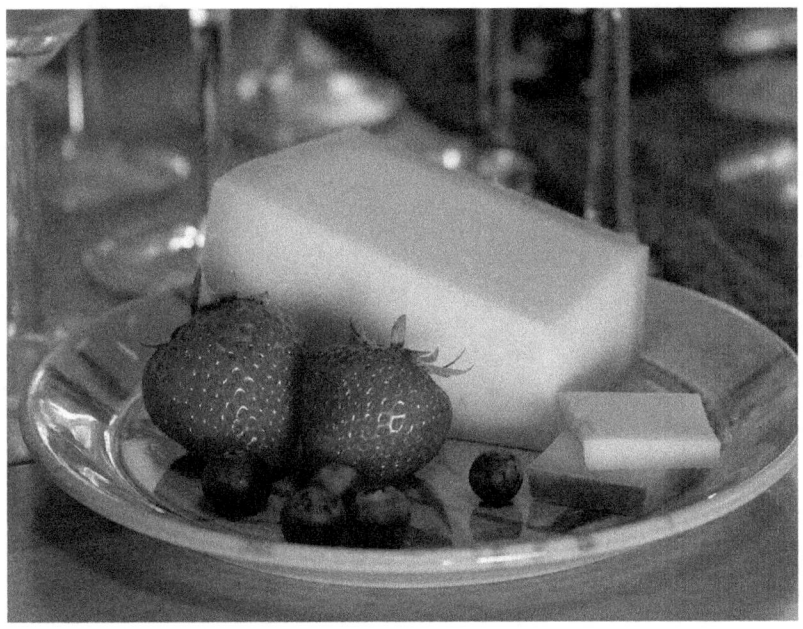

Customizing your diet according to your needs is essential to make the entire process effortless and enjoyable. You may take a look at the details below to figure out how you can make the DASH diet an ideal program for your taste and lifestyle.

Consider Your Favorite Foods

Listing your favorite foods is important in starting to make healthy food choices. If you like unhealthy foods such as pizza, hamburger, and junk foods, you can make certain modifications to improve your eating habits. You can use vegetable patty as a substitute to beef or cook a pizza that's less in sodium and processed meats. Bear in mind that you will have greater chances in giving up the diet if the foods you need to take are too unbearable for you. It's necessary that you are enjoying the healthy eating habits that you are trying to develop. This will help you resist temptations and continue the diet program.

Mix and Match Healthy Meals and Snacks

You also need to list down all the ingredients that you intend to consume in the diet. List down all the food items based on the type of vitamins and minerals that they contain. For instance, you can have a meal that's rich in potassium such as salmon and some dark leafy greens. You may then combine it with magnesium-rich fruits such as bananas and orange juice that are also rich in vitamin C and helps absorb calcium. Try to mix and match food items that you like to come up with a nutritionally balanced diet.

Choose Foods According to Your Goals

You should also customize your diet according to your goals. If you want to simply slim down and manage your weight, you can follow the ideal low-calorie DASH diet plan for weight loss. For instance, you can combine a variety of healthy foods and determine their overall calorie content. If you want to avoid or manage hypertension, you need to focus more on having low-sodium food choices and increase your intake on potassium, magnesium, and calcium. How you eat and the food choices you make should depend on a specific goal that you are trying to achieve.

State the Rules, Record, and Revise

You need to set your own rules in following the DASH diet, and you also need the will to pursue them to keep you from doing the things that you should avoid. Take, for instance, declaring that you will not eat at fast food chains or you will reduce and eventually eliminate consumption of processed and salty foods. This includes the favorite foods mentioned above that you need to modify to become healthy. You also need to track the progress that you have since the start of your diet. If you think that you need to change something in your diet, do it and try new ones.

Ask Help from a Registered Dietician

Asking help from a registered dietician is also necessary as it is one of the best ways to have a diet plan that is tailored to your lifestyle and individual needs. Dieticians can help you meet your basic nutritional needs and achieve your goals.

You can do anything you want to customize the program according to your needs. Just make sure that you are still sticking to the basic rules of DASH dieting while making the changes.

Conclusion

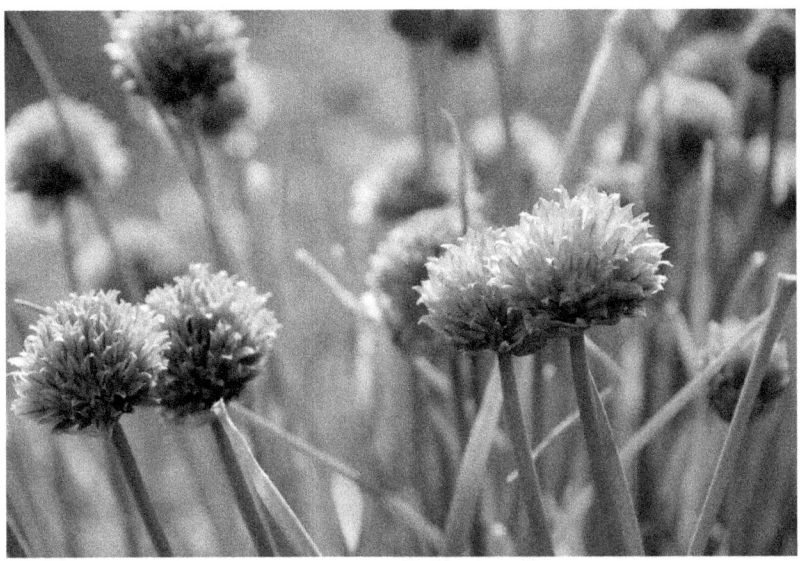

In following any diet, it is extremely essential that you put greater weight on satiety and not just the food choices that you make. Satiety is the feeling of satisfaction knowing that you have already consumed enough food. If you 're always satisfied with your daily diet, you will be eager to continue eating healthy foods. You need to make sure that you put a little twist to make your meals extremely interesting and tasty. This will help you stick to the diet program for a longer period.

Always bear in mind that you also need to engage in physical activities while dieting especially if you aim to lose weight. You need to start working out or doing something physical on a daily basis to make the diet more efficient. There are plenty of people who have benefited from following the diet. These people worked hard to improve their lifestyle and eating habits to achieve the healthy body and weight that they aim for.

There are different techniques to make the DASH diet a success. You can always make the diet a part of your daily life as well. It will keep you on the right track in correcting your unhealthy food preferences and in protecting yourself from various forms of medical conditions.

About the Author

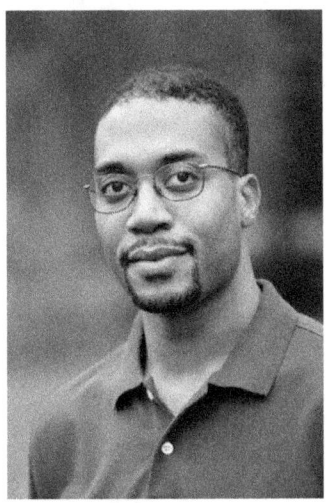

Dr. Terrell Clements was born and raised in Queens, New York. He attended the prestigious Johns Hopkins University choosing a specialization in Emergency Medicine.

Dr. Clements has lectured extensively to corporate and community groups on the importance of preventative care and healthy eating. Dr. Clements has always believed the relationship between doctor and patient contributes significantly to the overall quality of care and has built his career on this foundational belief.

Terrell and his wife enjoy quiet trips to the mountains and traveling the states in their RV.

Additional Resources

Top 10 Things You Need to Know About ObamaCare

Natural Allergy Remedies

A Simple Guide to Understanding Blood Pressure

How to Prevent & Reverse Diabetes

Goodbye Migraine: A Guide to Migraine Treatments & Remedies

Chill Out: Proven Ways to Reduce Stress

Eating Healthy: Superfoods to Beat Heart Disease

www.ingramcontent.com/pod-product-compliance
Lightning Source LLC
Chambersburg PA
CBHW060227290526
45789CB00003B/1441